35 Juicing Yummy Secrets

A Slimmer You in 30 days
With unbelievable weight loss

Guidelines to prepare the juice recipes.

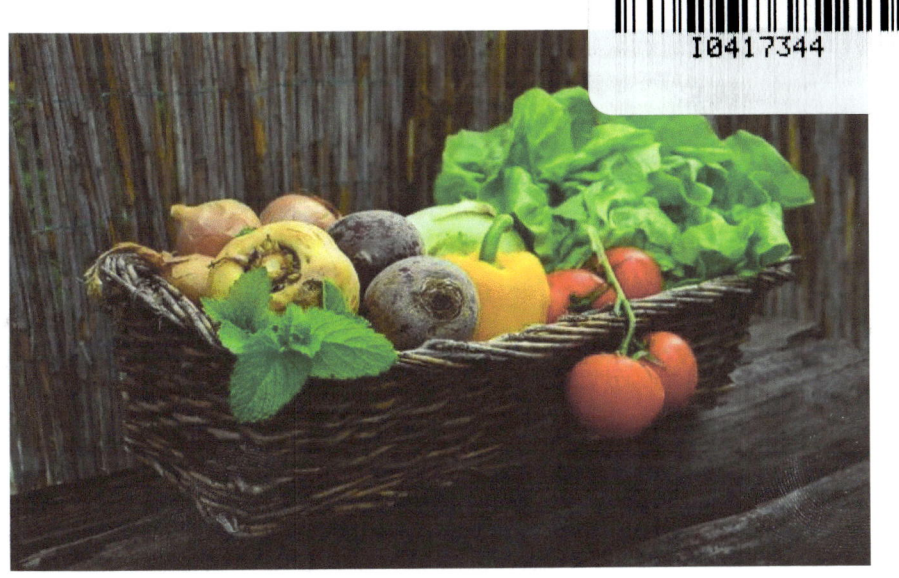

By: JANE HANSON

Legal & Disclaimer

The information contained in this book and its contents is not designed to replace or take the place of any form of medical or professional advice; and is not meant to replace the need for independent medical, financial, legal or other professional advice or services, as may be required. The content and information in this book has been provided for educational and entertainment purposes only.

The content and information contained in this book has been compiled from sources deemed reliable, and it is accurate to the best of the Author's knowledge, information and belief. However, the Author cannot guarantee its accuracy and validity and cannot be held liable for any errors and/or omissions. Further, changes are periodically made to this book as and when needed. Where appropriate and/or necessary, you must consult a professional (including but not limited to your doctor, attorney, financial advisor or such other professional advisor) before using any of the suggested remedies, techniques, or information in this book.

Upon using the contents and information contained in this book, you agree to hold harmless the Author from and against any damages, costs, and expenses, including any legal fees potentially resulting from the application of any of the information provided by this book. This disclaimer applies to any loss, damages or injury caused by the use and application, whether directly or indirectly, of any advice or information presented, whether for breach of contract, tort, negligence, personal injury, criminal intent, or under any other cause of action.

You agree to accept all risks of using the information presented inside this book.

You agree that by continuing to read this book, where appropriate and/or necessary, you shall consult a professional (including but not limited to your doctor, attorney, or financial advisor or such other advisor as needed) before using any of the suggested remedies, techniques, or information in this book.

Table of Contents

Introduction

Many dieting fads and methods come and go, but juicing for weight loss seems to be always there. It might just bob under the surface for a while, but it always reappears. It has proven itself over time, and people who try it usually become very devoted to it. Some of the juicing diet methods in circulation seem to have begun in Hollywood. For example, the pop singer, Beyoncé was once involved with a cayenne pepper and maple juice diet and even went on to endorse it. However, the proper, traditional method of juicing - by following a planned strategy to ensure your body is continuing to benefit from a full range of vitamins, proteins, minerals, and nutrients - is the one that works! It does what it says on the tin. It saturates your body with liquid sunshine, feeds the organs, bones, muscles and cells, makes you feel a gazillion dollars and most importantly melts those kilos away. If this is a dream, then I am living the dream!

When you follow a specific juicing (or half juicing which involves eating one low-calorie meal per day) plan, your body becomes saturated with vitamins, antioxidants, and nutrients, which will extract maximum performance from your body and help you to lose interest in sugary and salty snacks made of processed food.

 They are malnutrition and undigested food in the digestive tract. Juicing addresses the issue of malnutrition by satiating the body with vitamins, minerals, etc., and providing the correct nourishment that your body needs. Malnutrition sounds strange in the age of plenty, but when your body is subjected to a large dose of processed take away or supermarket foods, there is very little of nutritional value in these foods. Therefore your body is starved of nutrition and getting no benefit from these foods, hence the malnutrition. These foods are obviously tasty, but you would get the same nutrition from eating a piece of cardboard! In the cooking and pasteurizing or processing of these foods, nearly all the nutrition is destroyed.

Juicing also aids the colon's ability to rid itself of old debris that is stuck there - some of which may have been there for years! Juicing raw fruits and vegetables enable the body to heal and regenerate itself. Juicing helps progress the level of weight loss and fat burning by reducing cravings. I used to eat sweets and cakes by the bucket loads; nowadays I have no interest in them as the juice is providing me with the correct balance of nutrition. It also flushes out toxins and reduces acidity. As we get older, we find it more difficult to digest and fully absorb the nutrition in food. Fruits and vegetables are full of vitamins, minerals, anti-oxidants, and life enzymes that because they are juiced, they bypass the digestive system straight into our stomachs, then our blood stream, therefore ensuring that we get all the nutrition that we need. When the body has the necessary nutrition, it will perform better. Carrot is one example of an ingredient that should be in as many of our juices as possible, as they are very efficient at helping with fat burning. They are high in nutrients as well as vitamins B, C, D, E, K, and beta-carotene and stimulate the adrenal glands, which helps incite fat burning.

Cooking of food destroys enzymes. Enzymes are many in raw fruits and vegetables, and they are responsible for many chemical reactions in our body some of which support the metabolism of fats and carbohydrates. The enzymes have a vital function in keeping our nutrition to a maximum, and whereas they remain intact in raw food, cooking destroys most of them. Items, which improve digestion, are ginger, papaya, pineapple, mint, carrot and fennel. A digestive system that is not functioning efficiently is frequently linked with weight problems.

So on that note, try this divine recipe: 2 carrots, 1 parsnip, half a pineapple skin off, 2 apples, some ginger and 2 avocados. Juice everything except the Avocados. Remember to peel and remove the stone from avocados and they should be blended rather than juiced. Avocados and Bananas do not juice well and clog up the juicer, so always blend them. Find a nice tall glass, some ice, and Enjoy!

Losing weight need not be a tedious, unwelcomed chore. There is no need to miss meals or exercise until you drop. Try juicing and discover a better body-friendly way to drop those kilos easily.

Thank you for purchasing my book, it is my sincere hope it will answer your question on title weight loss.

1. Classic Simple Green Juice

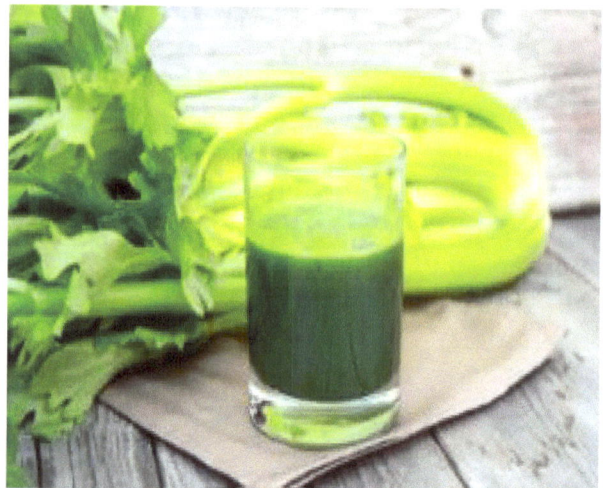

Nutritional Info: Calories: 184 Fat 0 g, Protein 1.5 g, Carbs 37

Servings: 1

Prep time: 10 minutes

Ingredients:

3 Apples

2 cups kale

2 stalks celery

One cup spinach¨

½ teaspoon spirulina

Directions:

1.   Remove core from the apples.
2.   Wash all the fruits and veggies.
3.   Juice the fruits and veggies and then stir to smooth out consistency and taste.
4.   Blend with the spiraling
5.   Served chilled.

2. Carrot Apple Ginger

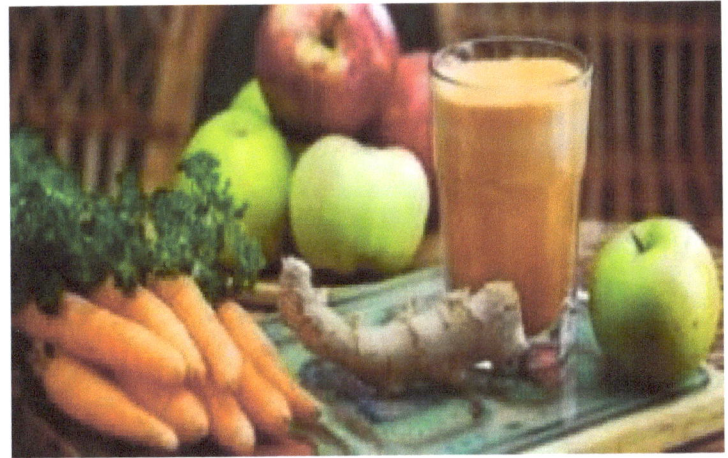

Nutritional Info: Calories: 156 Fat 0 g, Protein 1.5 g, Carbs 37

Servings: 1

Prep time: 10 minutes

Ingredients:

2 Apples

3 large carrots

One finger length of ginger root

Directions:

1.   Remove core from the apple.

2.   Wash all the fruits and veggies.

3.   Peel the ginger and optionally the carrots.

4.   Juice all ingredients and then stir to smooth out consistency and taste.

5.   Serve chilled

3.Pineapple Green Paradise

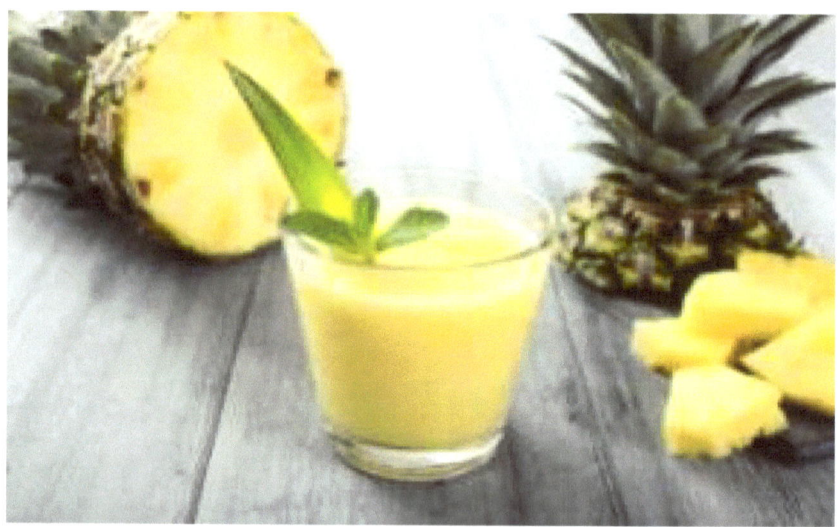

Nutritional Info: Calories: 195 Fat 0 g, Protein 1.5 g, Carbs 45

Servings: 1

Prep time: 10 minutes

Ingredients:

2 cups cubed pineapple

One half cucumber, cut into pieces small enough to easily fit in the juicer ½ cup coconut water

Directions:

1.   Wash the fruits and cucumber.

2.   Juice the pineapple and cucumber.

3.   Stir in the coconut water.

4.   Serve chilled.

4.Supreme Citrus

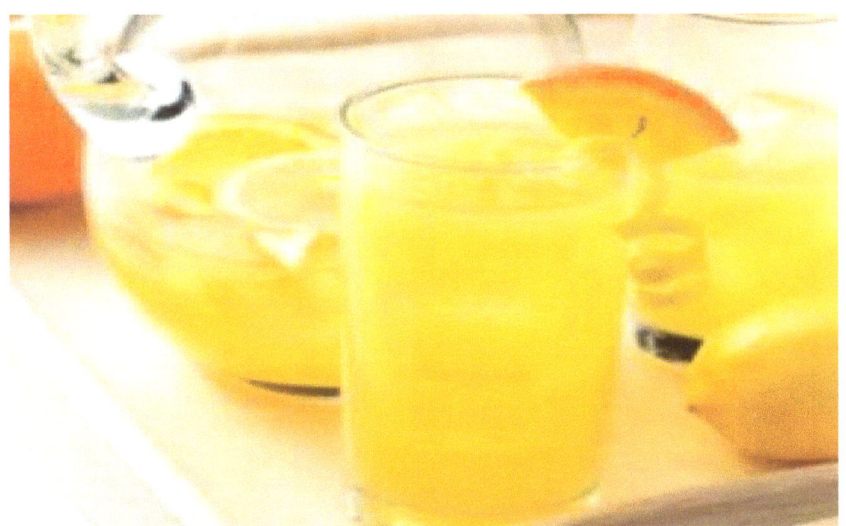

Nutritional Info: Calories: 215 Fat 0 g, Protein 0 g, Carbs 40

Servings: 1

Prep time: 10 minutes

Ingredients:

3 Oranges, peeled

1 lemon, peeled.

Directions:

1.   Rinse all the fruits.

2.   Juice the oranges and lemon.

3.   Stir the juice and place in the fridge.

4.   Serve chilled

5. Gimme Grapefruits

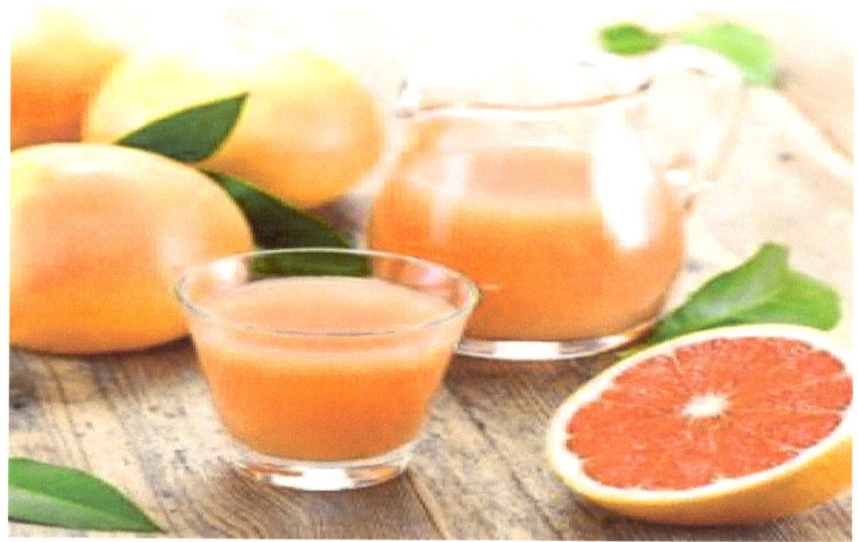

Nutritional Info: Calories: 215 Fat 0 g, Protein 0 g, Carbs 40

Servings: 1

Prep time: 10 minutes :

Ingredients:

2 Grapefruits, peeled

2 cups green grapes

Directions:

1.　　Rinse all the fruits.

2.　　Juice the grapefruits and grapes.

3.　　Stir the juice and place in the fridge.

4.　　Serve chilled

6. Strawberry Beet

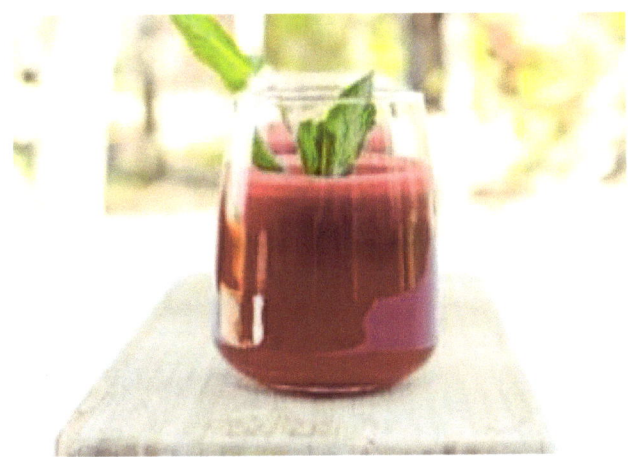

Nutritional Info: Calories: 215 Fat 0 g, Protein 0 g, Carbs 40

Servings: 1

Prep time: 10 minutes

Ingredients:

2 cups strawberries, stems removed

1 cup beets, peeled and chopped

½ cup coconut water

Directions:

1. Rinse all the fruits.

2. Juice the strawberries and beets.

3. Stir in the coconut water.

4. Stir the juice and place in the fridge.

5. Serve chilled.

7. Kiwi Cucumber

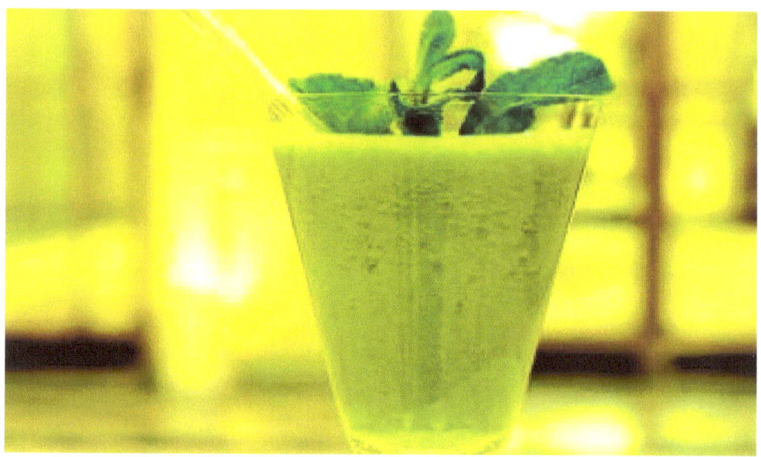

Nutritional Info: Calories: 176 Fat 0 g, Protein 0 g, Carbs 28

Servings: 1

Prep time: 10 minutes

Ingredients:

4 Kiwis, skin removed

One whole cucumber, sliced.

Directions:

1.   Rinse all the fruits and veggies.

2.   Juice the kiwi and cucumber.

3.   Stir the juice and place in the fridge.

4.   Serve chilled.

8. Blue Green

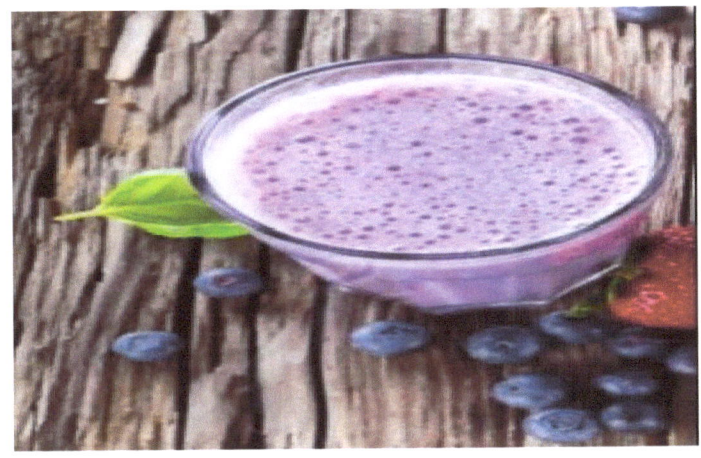

Nutritional Info: Calories: 154 Fat 0 g, Protein 0 g, Carbs 21

Servings: 1

Prep time: 10 minutes

Ingredients:

Two cups blueberries

One teaspoon cinnamon

One half a cucumber, chopped

One black plum, pit removed

Directions:

1. Rinse all the fruits and veggies.

2. Juice the blueberries, cucumber and plum.

3. Stir in the cinnamon or blend in a blender.

4. Stir the juice and place in the fridge.

5. Serve chilled.

9. The Best Red Juice

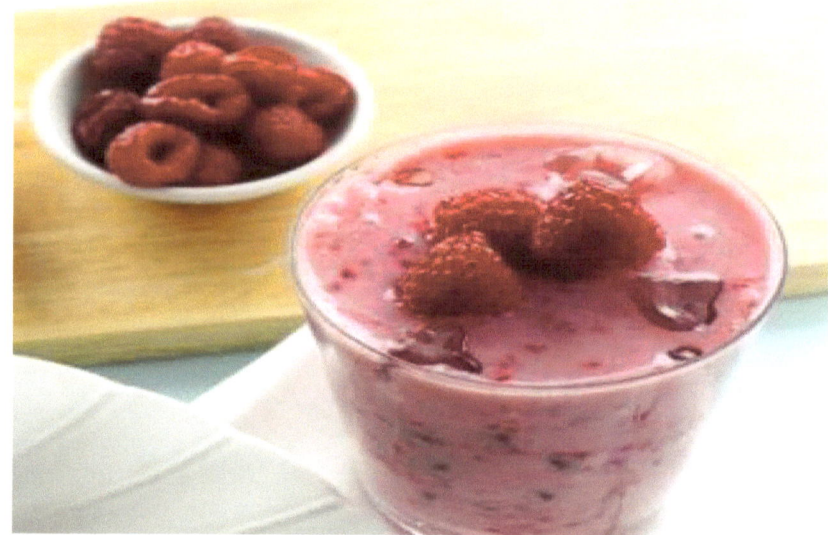

Nutritional Info: Calories: 215 Fat 0 g, Protein 0 g, Carbs 40

Servings: 1

Prep time: 10 minutes

Ingredients:

One cup strawberries, stems removed

One-cup raspberries

One apple, cored and chopped

½ cup red currants

Directions:

1.	Rinse all the fruits.

2.	Juice the fruits and berries.

3.	Stir the juice and place in the fridge.

4.	Serve chilled.

10. Orange Bliss

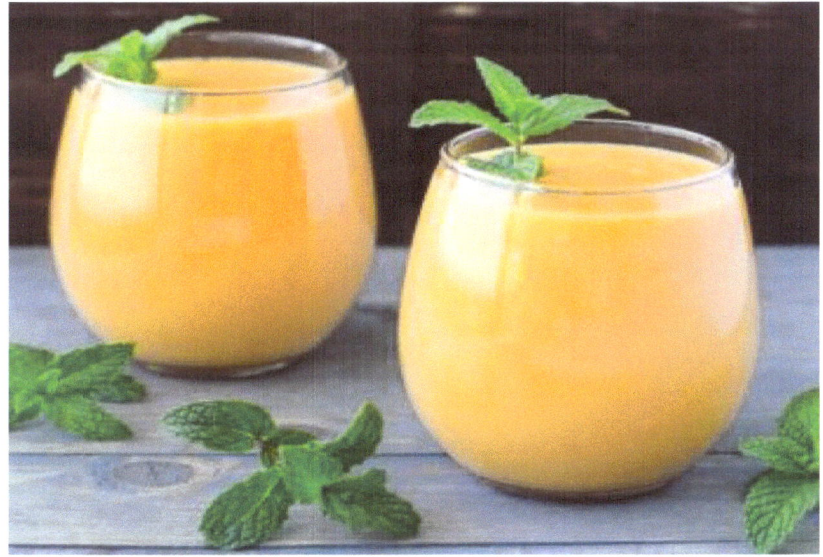

Nutritional Info: Calories: 240 Fat 0 g, Protein 0 g, Carbs 37

Servings: 1

Prep time: 7 minutes

Ingredients:

3 oranges, peeled

One-cup coconut water

Directions:

1. Juice the peeled oranges.

2. Stir in the coconut water

3. Place in fridge.

4. Serve chilled.

11. Yellow Heaven

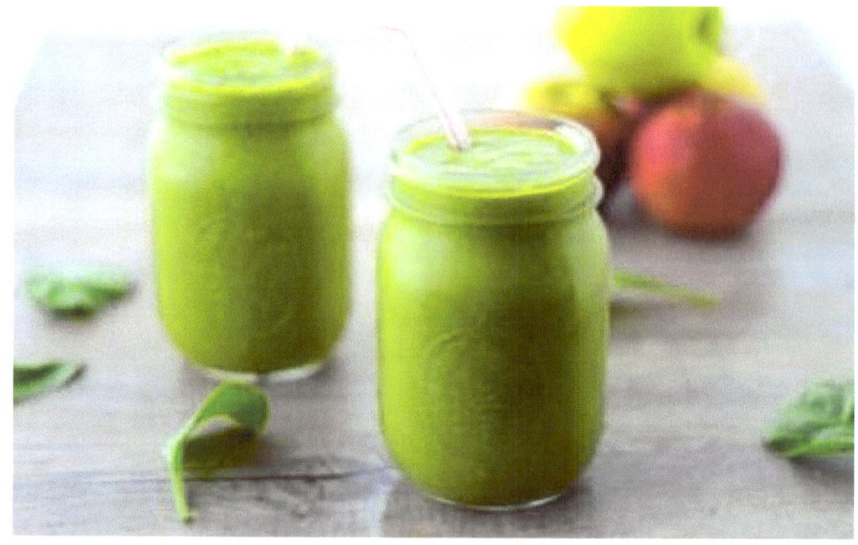

Nutritional Info: Calories: 240 Fat 0 g, Protein 0 g Carbs 40

Servings: 1

Prep time: 10 minutes

Ingredients:

2 lemons, with peel if organic

One finger length turmeric root

2 apples, cored

Directions:

1.   Rinse all the lemons, turmeric and apples

2.   Juice everything.

3.   Stir the juice and place in the fridge.

4.   Serve chilled.

12. Green Supreme

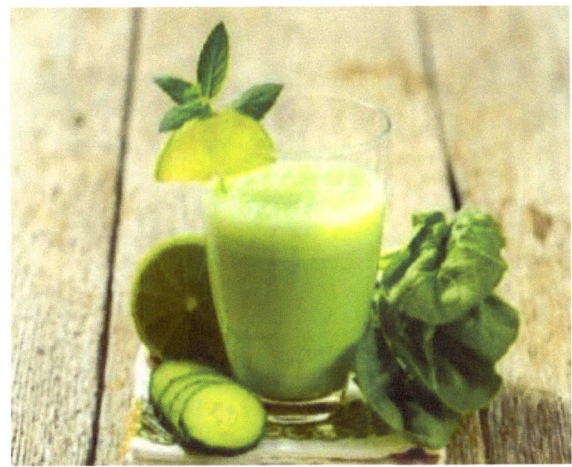

Nutritional Info: Calories: 240 Fat 0 g, Protein 0 g, Carbs 36

Servings: 1

Prep time: 10 minutes

Ingredients:

One-cup kale

One-cup spinach

One whole cucumber

1/2 teaspoon cinnamon

Two cups pineapple, cubed

Directions:

1.   Rinse off the fruit and veggies.

2.   Juice the kale, spinach, cucumber and pineapple.

3.   Stir in cinnamon and place in the fridge. Also may be enjoyed room temperature.

4.   Serve chilled.

13. Beautiful Blues

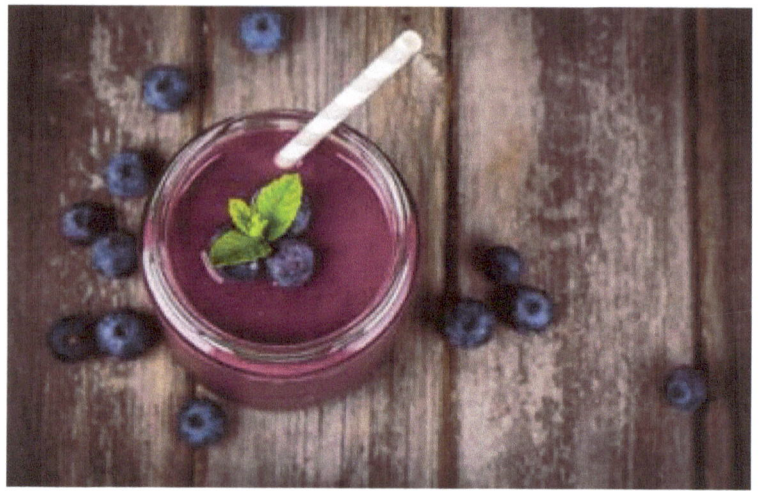

Nutritional Info: Calories: 250 Fat 0 g, Protein 0 g, Carbs 33

Servings: 1

Prep time: 10 minutes

Ingredients:

4 plums, pits removed

One cup black currants

One cup blackberries

½ cup blueberries

Directions:

1. Rinse all the fruits.

2. Juice the fruits.

3. Stir the juice and place in the fridge. Also may be enjoyed room temperature .

4. Serve chilled.

14. Natural Detox Juice

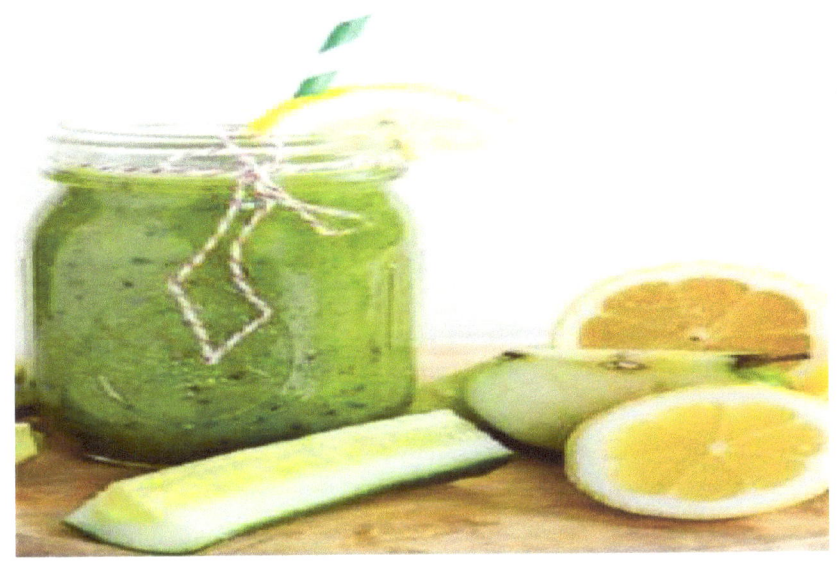

Nutritional Info: Calories: 190 Fat 0 g, Protein 0 g, Carbs 28

Servings: 1

Prep time: 10 minutes

Ingredients:

One finger length turmeric

One finger length ginger root

One organic lemon with peel on

One whole cucumber, sliced

One apple

One tablespoon apple cider vinegar

Directions:

1.   Rinse all the fruits and veggies.

2.   Juice the roots, lemon and cucumber.

3.   Stir in the apple cider vinegar.

4.   Stir the juice and place in the fridge. Also may be enjoyed room temperature .

5.   Serve chilled.

15. Anti-Inflammation

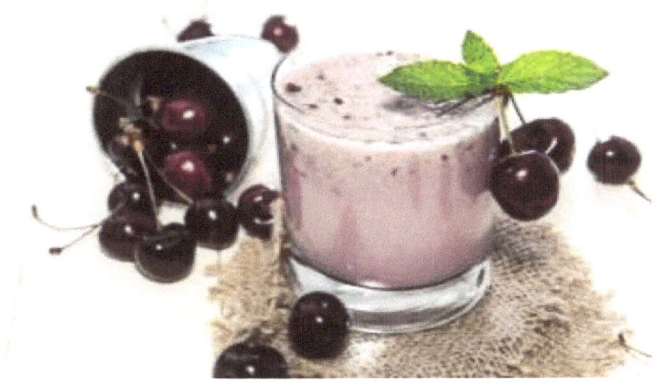

Nutritional Info: Calories: 190 Fat 0 g, Protein 0 g, Carbs 28

Servings: 1

Prep time: 10 minutes

Ingredients:

One finger length turmeric

One finger length ginger root

One-cup cherries, seeds removed

One apple, core removed

One pinch black pepper

Directions:

1.   Rinse the fruits and roots.

2.   Juice the roots, cherries and apple.

3.   Stir in the pepper.

4.   Stir the juice and place in the fridge. Also may be enjoyed room temperature

5.   Serve chilled.

16. Immunity

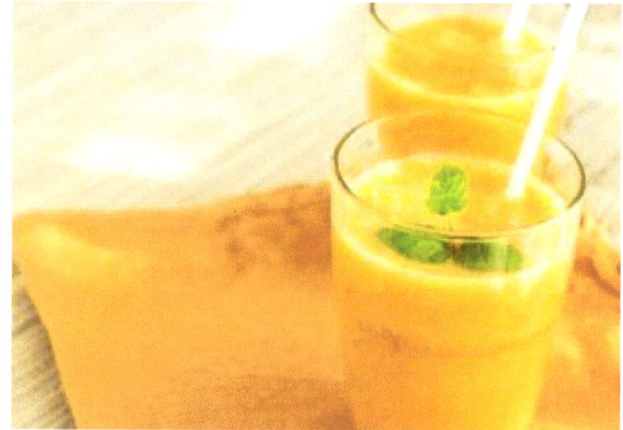

Nutritional Info: Calories: 207 Fat 0 g, Protein 0 g, Carbs 3

servings: 1

Prep time: 10 minutes

Ingredients:

2 oranges, peeled

One lemon, peel left on if organic

One finger length ginger root

Five drops oregano oil

½ teaspoon chilli powder

Directions:

1.   Rinse all the fruits and roots.

2.   Juice the roots, oranges and lemon.

3.   Stir in the oregano oil and chili powder.

4.   This spicy drink will help keep you healthy and to fight off colds.

5.   Serve at room temperature or chilled.

17. Garden Glory

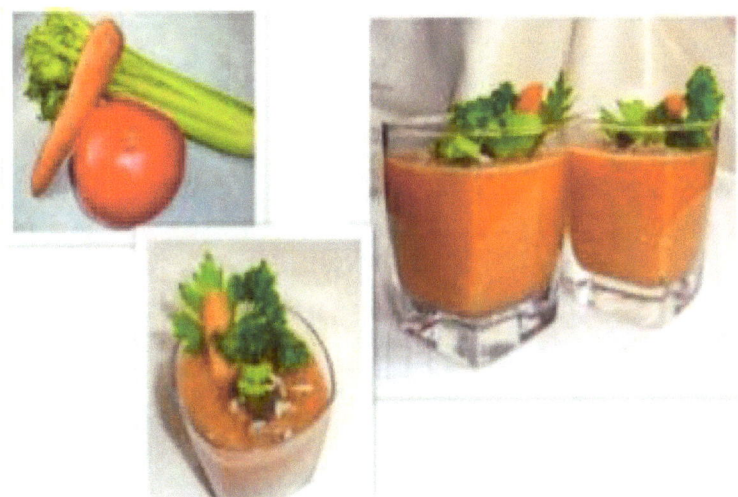

Nutritional Info: Calories: 183 Fat 0 g, Protein 0 g Carbs 22

Servings: 1

Prep time: 10 minutes

Ingredients:

One-cup spinach

One tomato, stem removed

Two carrots, peeled and cut

One stalk celery

Directions:

1.   Rinse all the veggies.

2.   Juice everything.

3.   Serve at room temperature or chilled.

18. Autumn Aurora

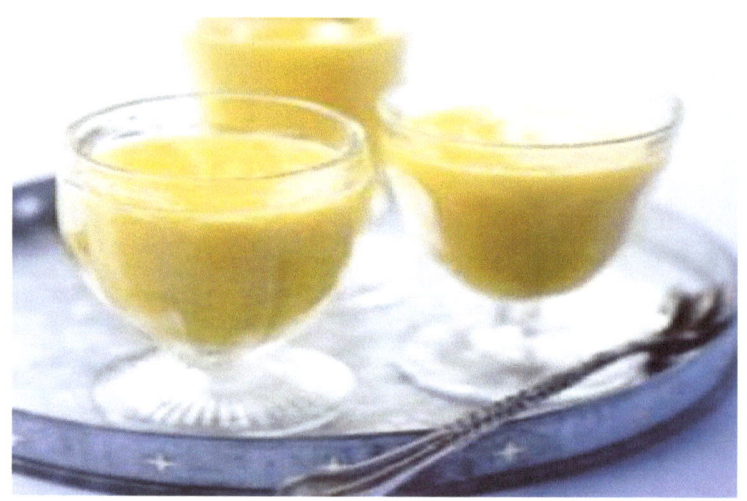

Nutritional Info: Calories: 250 Fat 0 g, Protein 0 g, Carbs 34

Servings : 1

Prep time: 10 minutes

Ingredients:

Two apples, cored

Two pears, cored

One-teaspoon cinnamon

Directions:

1.   Rinse all the fruits.

2.   Juice the apples and pears.

3.   Stir in the cinnamon.

4.   Stir the juice and place in the fridge.

5.   Serve chilled.

19. Winter Warmer

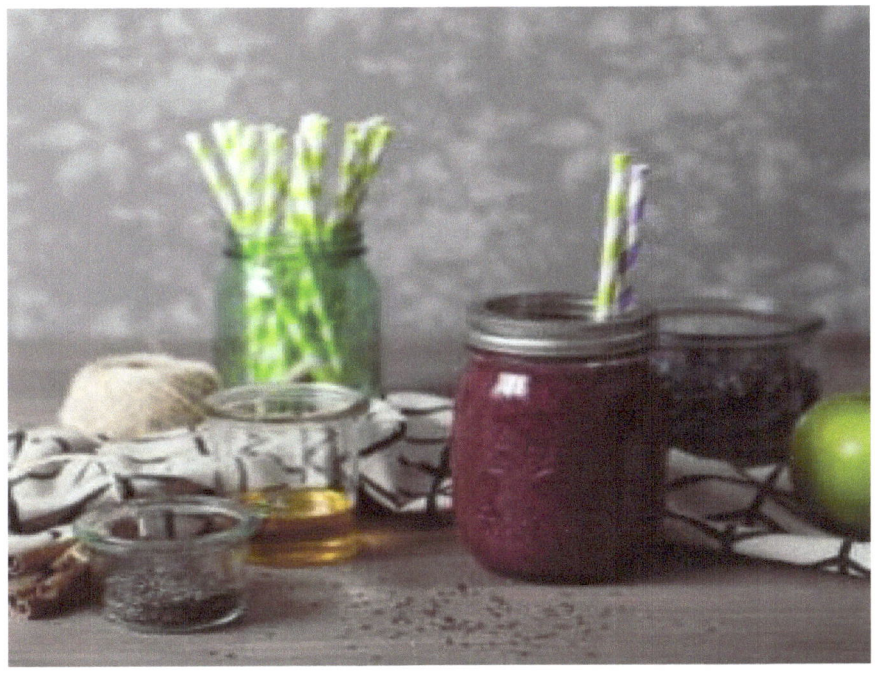

Nutritional Info: Calories: 260 Fat 0 g, Protein 0 g, Carbs 3

Servings: 1

Prep time: 10 minutes

Ingredients:

Two apples, cored

Two oranges

One cup cherries

One cup blueberries

¼ teaspoon ground cloves

One teaspoon cinnamon

½ teaspoon ginger powder

Directions:

1.   Rinse all the fruits.

2.   Juice the apples, oranges, cherries and blueberries.

3.   Stir in the cinnamon, cloves and ginger.

4.   Heat gently in a saucepan. Stir and serve warm in the wintertime.

5   Serve chilled if preferred.

20. Spring Clean

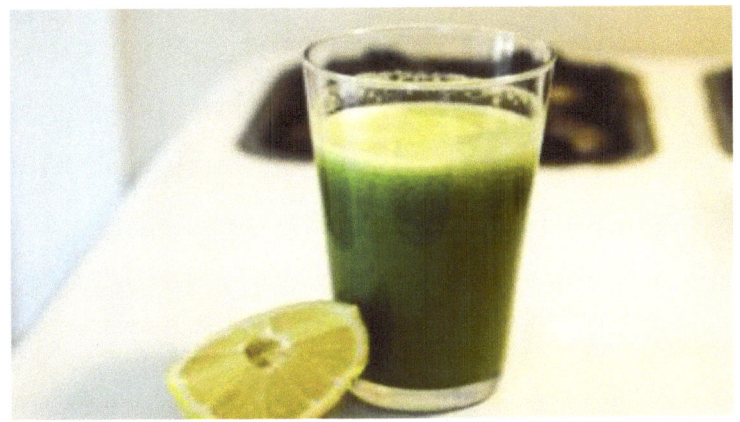

Nutritional Info: Calories: 223 Fat 0 g, Protein 0 g Carbs 29

Servings: 1

Prep time: 10 minutes

Ingredients:

Two lemons, peel left on if organic

Two finger length pieces of ginger

One cup spinach

One tablespoon maple syrup

Directions:

1. Rinse all the fruits, veggies and root.

2. Juice the lemons and the spinach and ginger.

3. Stir in the maple syrup.

4. Place in the refrigerator.

5. Serve chilled.

21. Pine Colada

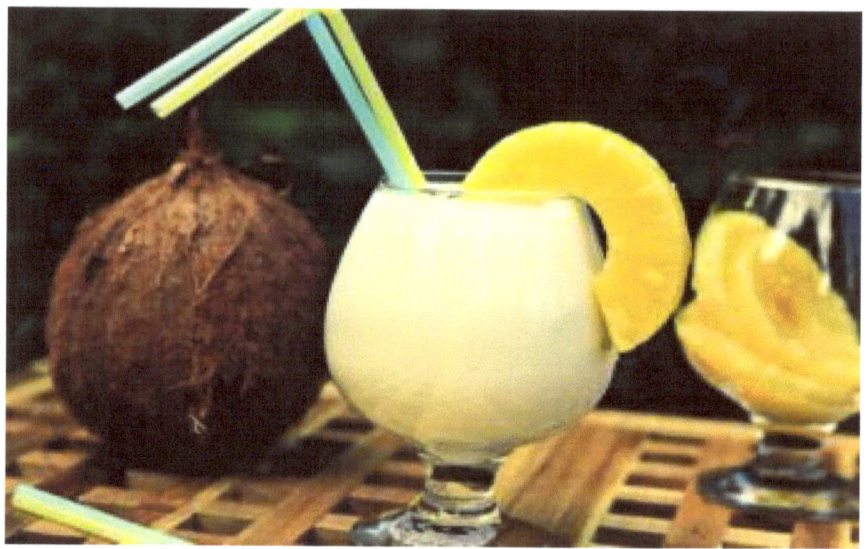

Nutritional Info: Calories: 215 Fat 7 g, Protein 0 g ,Carbs 27

Servings: 1

Prep time: 10 minutes

Ingredients:

Two cups pineapple

One cup coconut milk

Directions:

1.   Rinse off the fruit.

2.   Juice the pineapple.

3.   Blend the coconut milk and the pineapple.

4.   Serve with ice.

22. After Sport Pick Me Up

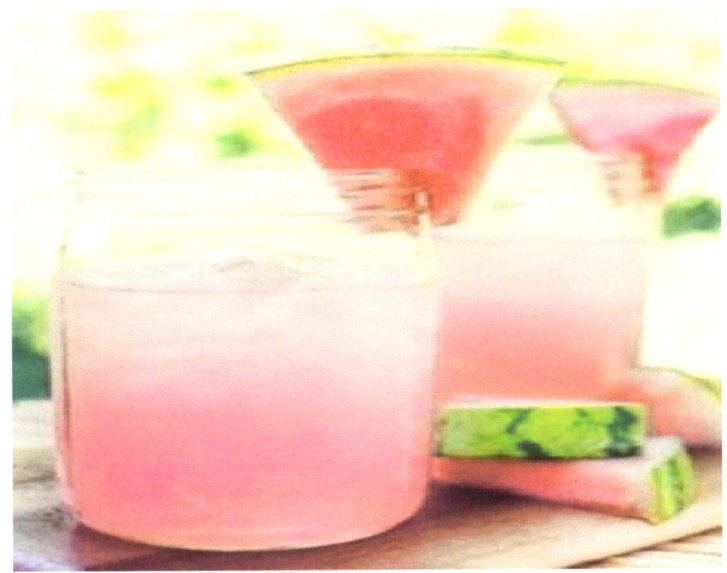

Nutritional Info: Calories: 170 Fat 0 g, Protein 0 g, Carbs 25

Servings: 1

Prep time: 10 minutes

Ingredients:

One cup watermelon

One cup coconut water

Directions:

1. Cut up the fruit.

2. Juice the watermelon.

3. Stir in the coconut water.

23. Strawberry Ginger Paradise

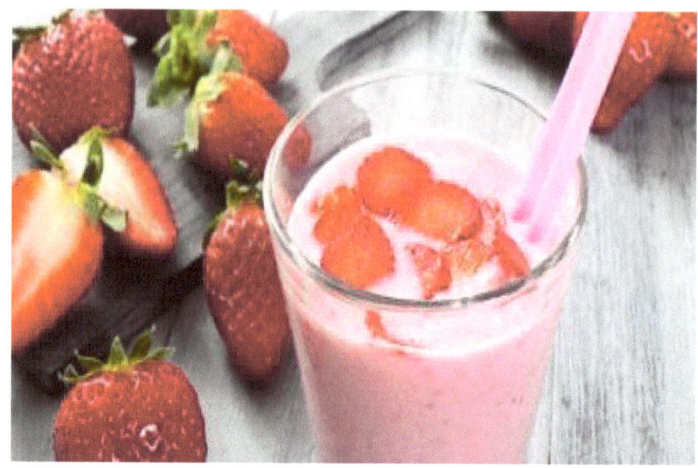

Nutritional Info: Calories: 225 Fat 7 g, Protein 0 g, Carbs 37

Servings : 1

Prep time: 10 minutes

Ingredients:

Two cups strawberries

One finger length ginger root

½-cup coconut milk

Directions:

1.   Rinse all the fruits and root.

2.   Juice the strawberries and the ginger root.

3.   Stir in the coconut milk.

4.   Serve at room temperature or chilled.

24. Blackberry Bramble

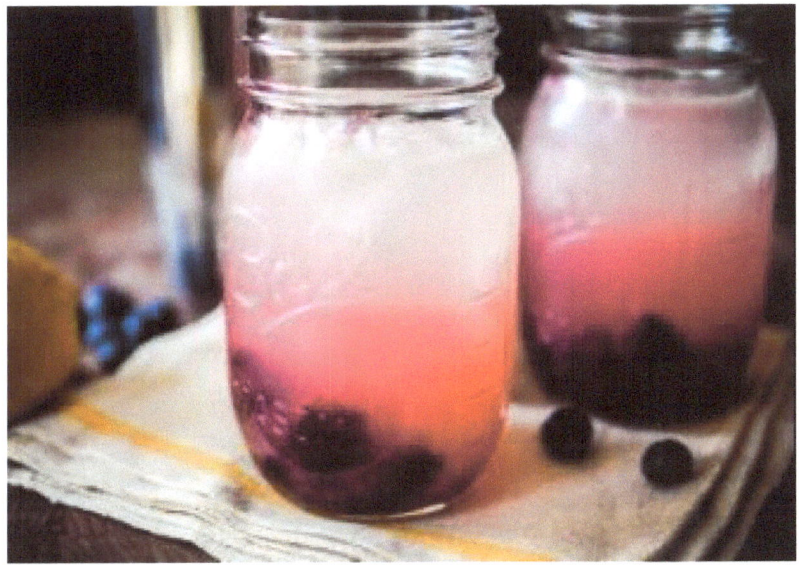

Nutritional Info: Calories: 189 Fat 0 g, Protein 0 g, Carbs 34

Servings: 1

Prep time: 10 minutes

Ingredients:

Two cups blackberries

One cup raspberries

One half apple, cored

Directions:

1. Rinse all the fruits.

2. Juice the blackberries, raspberries and apple.

3. Serve with ice .

25. Cherry Berry

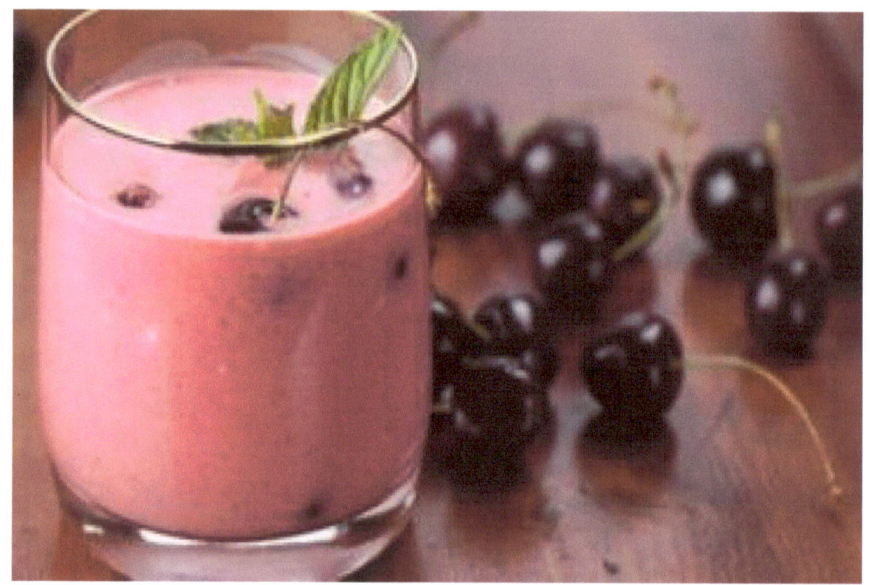

Nutritional Info: Calories: 219 Fat 0 g, Protein 0 g, Carbs 37

Servings: 1

Prep time: 10 minutes

Ingredients:

Two cups cherries, pits removed

One cup raspberries

½ cup strawberries

Directions:

1.   Rinse all the fruits.

2.   Juice the cherries, raspberries and strawberries.

3.   enjoy at room temperature.

26. Tomato Garden

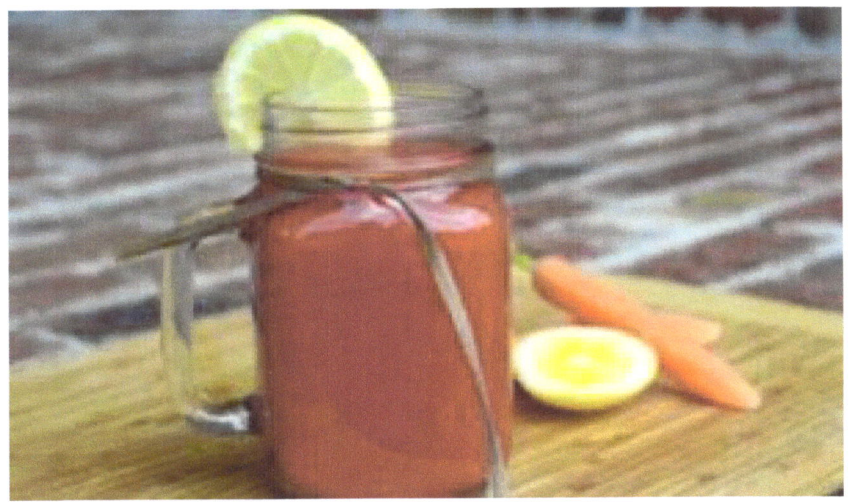

Nutritional Info: Calories: 210 Fat 0 g, Protein 0 g, Carbs 16

Servings: 1

Prep time: 10 minutes

Ingredients:

Two cups chopped tomato

Two carrots, peeled and chopped

One cup kale, peel left on if organic

Directions:

1.   Rinse all the veggies.

2.   Juice the tomato, carrots and kale.

3.   Serve with ice.

27. Elderberry Strengthener

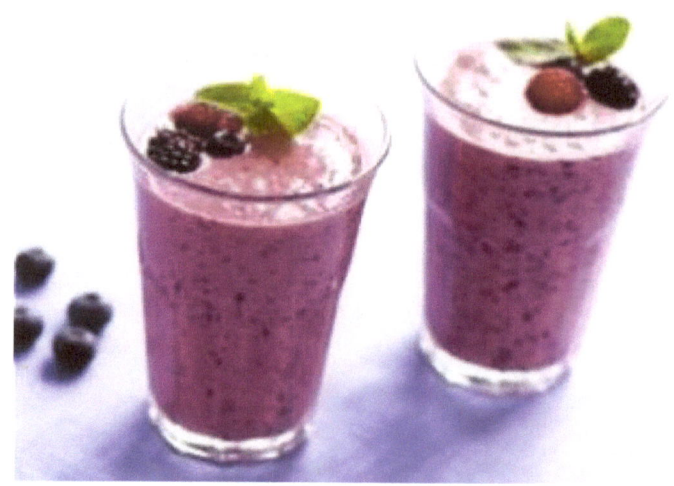

Nutritional Info: Calories: 215 Fat 0 g, Protein 0 g, Carbs 26

Servings: 1

Prep time: 10 minutes

Ingredients:

Two cups elderberries

One apple, cored, cut into pieces

One finger's length of ginger root

Directions:

1.   Rinse all the fruits and root.

2.   Juice the elderberries, apple and ginger.

3.   Serve with ice. Elderberries strengthen the immune system and digestion.

28. Merlot Juice

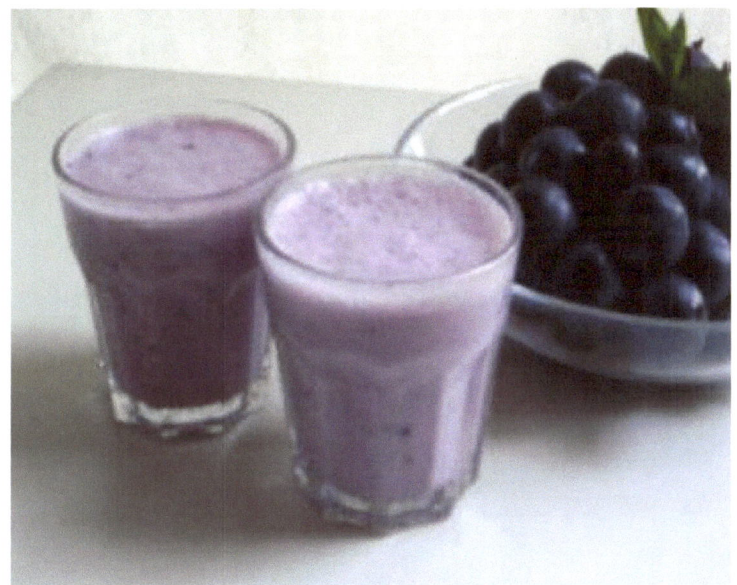

Nutritional Info: Calories: 80 Fat 0 g, Protein 0 g, Carbs 18

Servings: 1

Prep time: 10 minutes

Ingredients:

Two cups merlot grapes

½-cup sparkling water

Directions:

1.　　Rinse all the grapes.

2.　　Juice the grapes.

3.　　Stir in the sparkling water

4.　　Serve with ice.

29. Sweet Potato Pear Juice

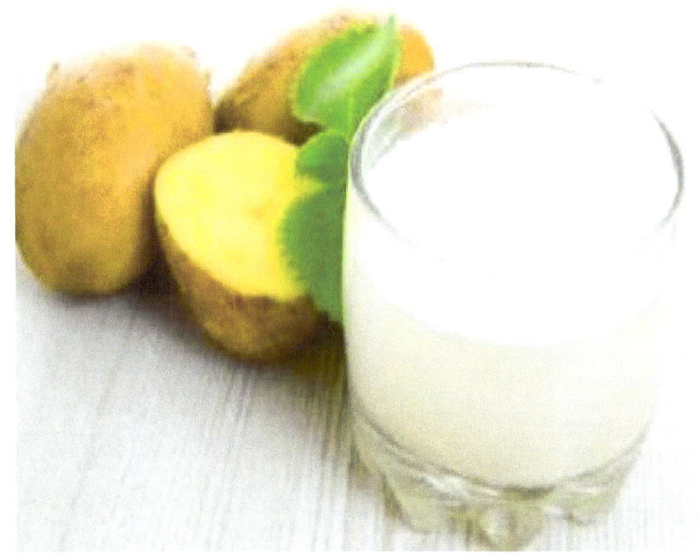

Nutritional Info: Calories: 305 Fat 6 g, Protein 0 g, Carbs 45

Servings: 1

Prep time: 10 minutes

Ingredients:

Two cups chopped sweet potato

Three pears, core removed and chopped One cup coconut milk

Directions:

1.   Rinse all the sweet potatoes and pears.

2.   Juice the sweet potatoes and pears.

3.   Stir in the coconut milk.

4.   Serve at room temperature.

30. Kaki Fruit Deliciousness

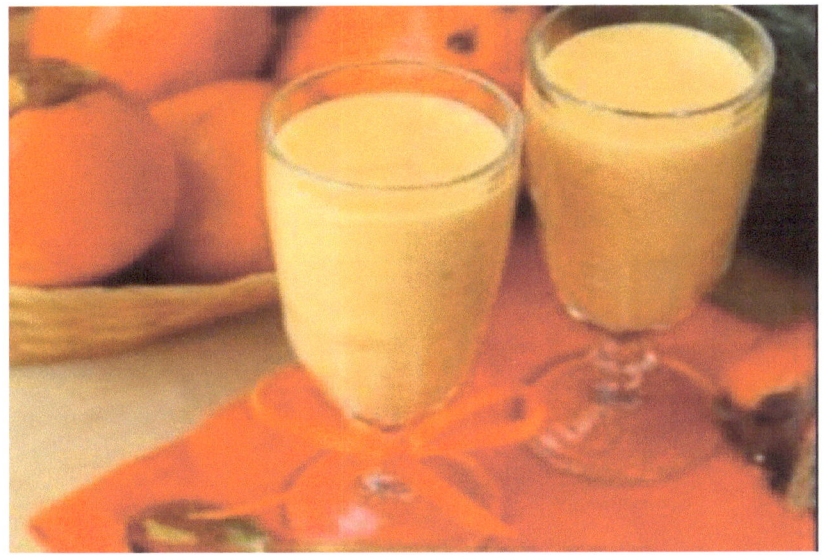

Nutritional Info: Calories: 263 Fat 0 g, Protein 0 g, Carbs 47

Servings: 1

Prep time: 10 minutes

Ingredients:

Four kaki fruits, skin removed

One orange, peeled

Directions:

1.   Rinse all the fruits.

2.   Juice the kaki fruits and orange.

3.   Serve at room temperature.

31. Exotic Litchi Delight

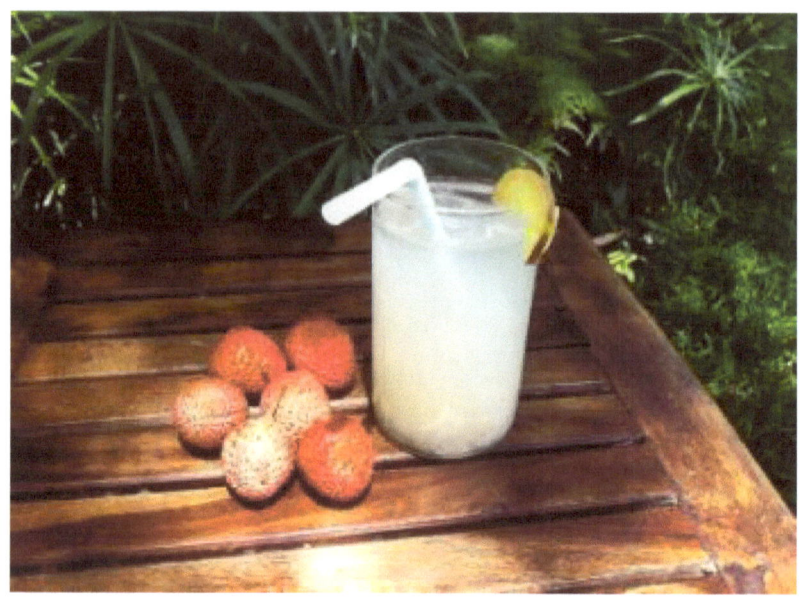

Nutritional Info: Calories: 189 Fat 0 g, Protein 0 g Carbs 33

Servings : 1

Prep time: 10 minutes

Ingredients:

Three cups litchi fruits, pits removed and outer shell removed

One cup coconut water

Directions:

1.   Rinse all the litchi fruits.

2.   Juice the litchis.

3.   Stir in the coconut water.

4.   Serve chilled.

32. Star Fruit Dragon Fruit Cosmic Juice

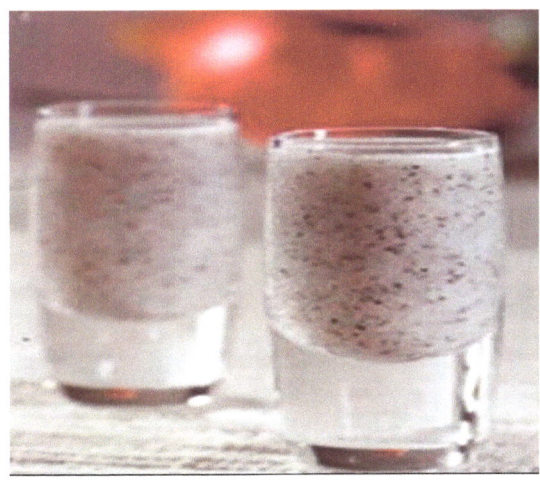

Nutritional Info: Calories: 120 Fat 0 g, Protein 0 g, Carbs 29

Servings: 1

Prep time: 10 minutes

Ingredients:

One dragon fruit, skin removed and cut into small pieces

Two star fruits, skin removed, chopped

One cup coconut water

Directions:

1.   Rinse all the fruits.

2.   Juice the star fruits and dragon fruit.

3.   Stir in the coconut water.

4.   Serve at room temperature.

33. Orange Banana Tropics

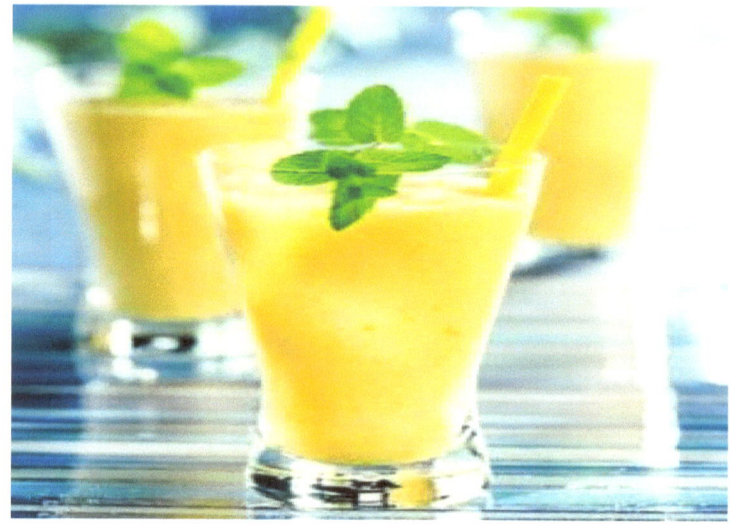

Nutritional Info: Calories: 200 Fat .5 g, Protein 0 g, Carbs 43

Servings: 1

Prep time: 10 minutes

Ingredients:

Two oranges, peeled

One banana, peeled

One cup coconut water

Directions:

1.   Rinse all the oranges.

2.   Juice the oranges.

3.   Place the orange juice along with the banana and the coconut water in a blender.

4.   Blend and serve at room temperature, or chill in the fridge.

34. Raspberry Coconut Swirl

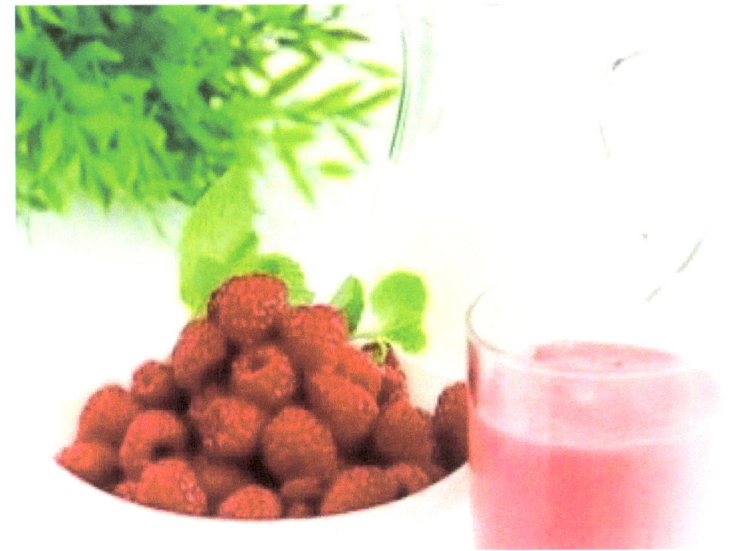

Nutritional Info: Calories: 280 Fat 7 g, Protein 0 g, Carbs 40

Servings: 1

Prep time: 10 minutes

Ingredients:

Three cups raspberries

One cup coconut milk

One cup coconut water

Directions:

1.   Rinse all the raspberries.

2.   Stir in the coconut milk and coconut water.

3.   Serve at room temperature and enjoy.

35. Orange Lemon Banana

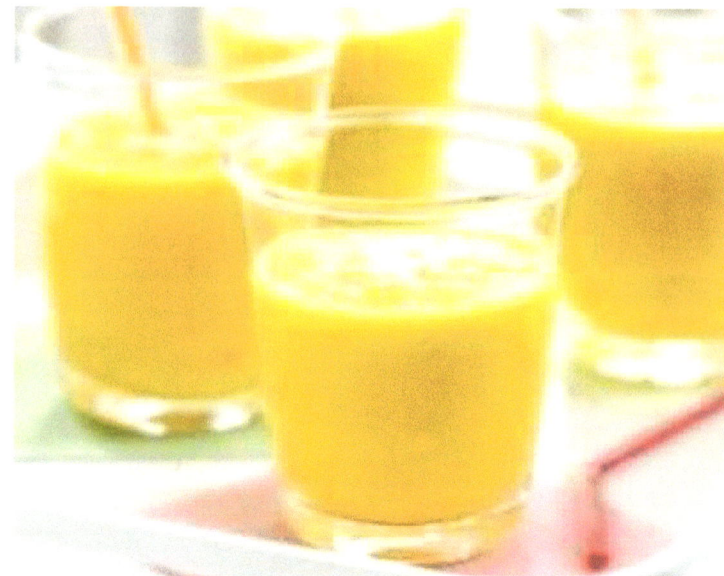

Nutritional Info: Calories: 287 Fat 7 g, Protein 0 g, Carbs 40

Servings: 1

Prep time: 10 minutes

Ingredients:

One Orange, peeled

Two lemons, peeled

One finger ginger

One banana, peeled

Directions:

1. Divide the oranges into pieces and cut the lemons.

2. Juice the oranges and lemon.

3. Juice the ginger.

4. Place the juice in the blender with the banana.

5. Blend and serve chilled.

Conclusion

I hope this book was able to help you in understanding the different benefits healthy juices have got to offer. If you are on a diet and you want to lose a couple of inches without depriving your body of essential nutrients, then you can make use of these healthy and tasty juicing recipes for achieving your goal. You will not only be losing weight but you will also be able to make sure that you stay healthy.

The next step is to simply gather all the necessary ingredients and get started with following the recipes to recreate simple and tasty juices that will help you in achieving your health and weight goals. Shopping for the necessary ingredients will not take you long because of the detailed list of ingredients that have been provided in the book along with the recipes. You cannot only follow the recipes that have been mentioned in the book but you can also come up with a variation of these recipes. Now that you are equipped with the knowledge regarding the nutritional aspects of various fruits and vegetables, you can experiment and come up with different delicious juices and smoothies. The next time you find yourself craving for something sweet or you just feel like indulging in an evening snack, then instead of grabbing a sugary and starchy snack, you can whip up one of the simple juicing recipes given in this book.

Thank you for purchasing this book, I hope you will apply the acquired knowledge productively.

www.ingramcontent.com/pod-product-compliance
Lightning Source LLC
Chambersburg PA
CBHW050839290526
45792CB00001B/460